10-Day Green Smoothie Cleanse

The Healthy Way To Lose Weight Incredibly Fast!

Table of Contents

Introduction

Are you yearning to lose weight fast? Do you want to do something about your weight now? Are you tired of taking too long to lose weight? While I know losing weight over a long period is what is advisable, there are moments when you just want to lose weight fast and you don't have several months to do that. If this is your case, then you have come to the right place.

The 10 day green smoothie cleanse will enable you to achieve your dreams fast. Actually, it is the ultimate secret to shedding most pounds within the shortest time possible. You will learn what to do during the cleanse, what not to eat as well as some helpful tips to help you deal with detox symptoms. Do not worry about the pounds rushing back in; we will also look at ways to make sure that you keep off the pounds.

What is the 10-Day Green Smoothie Cleanse

You must be wondering what this is all about apart from the fancy name. The 10 day green smoothie cleanse is a detox program where you eat green leafy vegetables, fruits and water for 10 days. This is designed to make sure that you lose weight fast before getting to the maintenance phase where you will work on maintaining the attained weight. According to this plan, the first step in losing weight is detoxification. The toxins are said to be harbored in the fat cells and are very difficult to get rid of. Examples of toxins that can be found outside your body are pesticides, cigarette smoke and other pollutants. Toxins inside our bodies are in form of viruses, bacteria, fungi, heavy metals among others that can cause cancer. The great thing about this weight loss program is that it focuses on both fat loss and detoxification ultimately improving your health and wellbeing. So, what does detoxification in this case mean? You detoxify by eliminating certain types of foods for 10 days. After the 10 days, your body will be used to eating the healthy food full of nutrients. Therefore, it will naturally crave and desire the healthy natural food. Seems hard to believe but those who have been through it successfully, have the same story to tell. Why don't we also make the story yours to tell?

But before we look at the details on this cleanse, it is important to know how you stand to benefit.

Health Improvements After The Cleanse

The beauty with the 10 day green smoothie cleanse is the benefits and health improvements that come with it. After the cleanse you can expect;

• Better sleep
• Less bloating
• Mental clarity
• Better digestion

- Increased energy
- Reduced cravings
- Weight loss

One of the things that the regular weight loss diets overlook is the presence of toxins in the body. This 10-day plan focuses on detoxification making it easier to achieve all of the above. Our body has the ability to eliminate the toxins but when it can't, then it stores them in the fat cells. There are different mechanisms by which toxins are eliminated. One of the ways is through the digestive system when we excrete. The other way is through the urinary system where the kidney filters out the body wastes. Another important system is the lymphatic system that collects the toxins from the blood vessels. The Integumentary system also plays a major role in toxin clearance especially through sweating. Owing to the large levels of toxins, the fat cells continue to expand and they literally weigh down the body and make it heavier leading to the systems becoming unable to function properly. As the toxins keep on accumulating, we start experiencing diseases like allergies, migraines, other other major diseases and at times general fatigue. Your body uses fat cells to bind the different toxins in order to prevent them from damaging the healthy cells. So in essence, the fats you've accumulated over the years are your friend since they help protect your body cells against harm from the toxins. As such, if you want to lose weight, the only workable solution to jumpstarting your weight loss journey is by eliminating the toxins first.

How The 10-Day Green Smoothie Cleanse Is Done

It is not as complex as you might have imagined it to be and it is quite easy to follow but only if you are determined. To fully have the health transforming experience;

• You will have to drink up to 60 ounces of green smoothies each day. Start by preparing your days smoothies either early in the morning or the previous day and make sure you keep it refrigerated. Take a third of it every three to 4 hours just as you would do your normal meals and snacks. Always sip on the smoothie when you feel hungry.

• You can also snack on fruits like apples, celery, carrots, cucumbers, and other crunchy vegetables. Something else that you could include in your diet are high protein foods like unsweetened peanut butter, raw and unsalted (only a handful) and also hard boiled eggs.

• Drink at least 8 glasses of water per day. Apart from this, you could also indulge in herbal teas.

• The foods that you will have to avoid completely are meat, cheese, refined sugar, refined carbs (white breads, pasta, doughnuts), processed and fried foods, liquor, coffee, beer, sodas and diet sodas.

Why Green Smoothie Cleanse

The question that must be lingering in your head is; why green smoothies? Given the fact that there are hundreds of diet plans, what would drive you into specifically choosing this one? Here are the 10 good reasons why green smoothie cleanse is something you want to try:

1. Weight loss; the first and most important reason is weight loss. The green smoothies might just be the best way to do it. This is especially because apart from the smoothies being high in nutrients, they are high in fiber that will give you a feeling of fullness the whole day without subjecting you to the risk of gaining weight. They also have a high water content, something that your body is in dire need of for detoxification. Water also makes you fuller.

2. Detoxification; it is very true that the body already has mechanisms in place to ensure that it gets rid of the toxins itself.

The problem is that with continued exposure, the mechanisms start failing too hence the accumulation of toxins in the fat cells. After the body utilizes the nutrients from the food that you have eaten, it must dispose off the unused particles. If the mechanisms for this are faulty then the body ends up absorbing these particles, which are toxins. The green smoothies come in handy since they are rich in fiber. They help the body to eliminate the toxins efficiently.

3. Nutrient rich: This is the other important bit about green smoothies. Most of the other foods have to be cooked hence subjecting them to high temperatures that damage the nutrients. This is not the case with the green smoothies; they are raw and very nutritious. They are full of vitamins, antioxidants, minerals, anti-inflammatory substances, phytonutrients, fiber, and water; the list is endless. Drinking the smoothies is like receiving a body cleansing transfusion.

4. Easy to digest; the fact that they have been blended and are in liquid form makes it very easy to digest. Most of us eat a lot of vegetables and fruits. They come in form of solids. At times, our body is not able to metabolize these foods efficiently. The smoothies come in a much pleasant form with the nutrients made readily available; hence, digestion is much easier.

5. Hydration; staying well-hydrated keeps the body healthy and energetic. It makes sure that your brain, your muscles, your immune system and your digestive system are all working perfectly. The green smoothies are high in water content and help you stay hydrated. Something else that you are supposed to do in the diet plan is take a lot of water. Most of us do not like the taste of water. In that case, all you can do is add a drop of lemon to improve the taste. When on the diet, you avoid taking things like cigarette, coffee, and soda. These are some of the causes of dehydration. It is very easy to tell if you are dehydrated just by checking your urine.

When dehydrated, your urine has a strong yellow color and stinks too compared to if you are not dehydrated.

6. Easy to make; it only takes you at most five minutes to finish preparing the green smoothies. All you need to do is sort out your ingredients at night. When you wake up, all you have to do is place them in the blender. After you are done, you clean up the blender, which is usually never messy, as compared to juicing and you are good to go.

7. Delicious; the green smoothies are a combination of healthy delicious fruits and vegetables. It is something that you would always love to sip on. The green color usually scares many people but once you learn to put the right combination of fruits and vegetables then you have nothing to worry.

8. Improved digestion; think about all the annoying indigestion problems that you always encounter; if you are not having a

bloated stomach then you are passing a lot of flatus. If it isn't the epigastric pain making you uncomfortable then it's the acid reflux. It is one problem after another. Now imagine living free of those problems; is it not amazing? Smoothies can give you the rest from all the stomach problems you are having. Smoothies are usually well blended and smooth; hence, they are not too hard to digest.

9. Vibrant, radiant health; this is easy to achieve when all you have is the good things mentioned above. With the healthy diet, all the systems in the body work for you from the first system that people encounter which is the skin. You end up looking younger and healthier glowing all the time. Your skin becomes supple and your acne disappears. Automatically your eyes become brighter and sparkle as the yellowness goes away. On the inside, your cells also rejuvenate making sure that all your organs work effectively and efficiently.

Tips For Success

I find it necessary to share some tips with you before you fully get into the diet plan. These tips will ensure that your journey is a little easier with more chances of success;

• Make a point of getting yourself a good and strong blender. If you have a good one then your blending time will only be 30 seconds, and all the ingredients will be nicely chopped leading to a nice creamy smooth smoothie. However if you have a low quality blender then you will have to double the time to 1 or 2 minutes. The end product is expected to be creamy and smooth.

• Make it taste good; for you to have an easier time with the smoothies, you will have to ensure that it does taste good. To achieve this, you can add more fruits, ice, or water. You can feel free to add a sweetener like Stevia. Make sure it works for you so that you are able to complete the cleanse. The experience does not have to be horrible.

• Make sure you add a scoop of protein to your smoothie. The protein will help make you full for longer and help with your metabolism. However, the protein can make the smoothie a little pasty so it is important to make a smoothie without it, then add some protein and see if you can tolerate. Avoid dairy protein and make use of the ones that we mentioned above.

• Drink plenty of water; we talked about drinking plenty of water. Ideally, you are supposed to drink 64 ounces of water. The advantage of taking a lot of water is that you will urinate frequently, which helps with cleansing your system.

• Drink herbal and detox tea; herbal tea helps in cleansing since they are usually high in antioxidants. Taking tea will also make you feel less hungry. Examples of good herbal teas include chamomile, green tea, peppermint, ginger, milk thistle, dandelion root, sarsaparilla and ginseng. You are free to add Stevia to taste.

• Chew your smoothies; the green smoothies are usually fine enough for you to just swallow without giving it time to be in your mouth. Although it may be difficult, try to chew your smoothies too. Remember that digestion starts from the mouth and we do not want to skip that stage. So keep it in your mouth for a little while.

• Rotate your greens; you will get to find out that all the greens have different alkaloids in them when we get to discuss the greens. It is therefore mandatory that, you alter them from week to week to avoid the accumulation of one type of alkaloid. If not it might lead to undesirable health effects.

• Expect weight fluctuation; I am sure this is the sad news but at least I did forewarn you. Your weight is bound to fluctuate. This is due to the muscles, fat, and water. The variation of the water content may contribute to the fluctuation. There is also the aspect of incorporating exercises that build up the muscle. When this happens, you gain some weight but remember in time you also burn some fat hence losing some more weight. You do not have to worry; a little fluctuation is allowed.

• Use ripe fruits; ripe fruits are sweeter and contain live enzymes that can be easily digested.

• Use frozen fruits; frozen fruits are cheaper and have just as much nutritional value as the fresh ones. It is therefore more convenient to use them. The other advantage is that they do not get spoilt. Fresh fruits have a tendency of going bad within a short time.

• Go easy on the fruit; add the fruits to taste but do not over do it. When you introduce too much sugar into the system, then you are going to have episodes of headaches. Just use some little fruit for the greens to taste. Try a new different fruit everyday because they alter the taste of green smoothies and it is this variation that will ensure you are not bored.

• Remove the stems from your greens; this depends on where you buy your greens. Some are bought already destemmed while some have the stems. The stems in the greens alter the taste of the smoothie and it might no longer be that desirable; hence, the reason it is advisable to remove the stems

• Do not starve yourself; do not confuse this with a starvation diet. When you are hungry, you are allowed to snack. The high protein snacks that we mentioned are the best so make a point of having them with you.

• Prepare to be uncomfortable; in the first days of the diet, you are bound to feel very hungry and irritable and as I said before, you are allowed to snack. Keep in mind though, that you cannot snack for the whole day, as you will end up losing no weight. It is okay to allow you body to be uncomfortable from time to time as it is only through this that you will get to train it to incorporate the healthy habits. After sometime, it is no longer going to be a problem so it also calls for your perseverance.

• Focus on getting healthy and the weight loss will follow; the good thing about this diet plan is the nutritional value. You can always remember that what you are doing is the right thing for the body and weight loss is just one of the good by products in the whole process.

• Build a green smoothie recipe box; there will be so many recipes that you will come across and try out. However, we are different and fancy different things. Make a point of writing down the green recipes that you tried out and liked so that you have a list of the favorite smoothies. This will make life easier and interesting for you.

• For the diabetics, you can purpose to use the low sugar fruits because of your concerns about your sugar levels. Examples of these fruits are grapes, apples, cherries, strawberries, goji berries, blueberries, raspberries, cranberries, lemons, and lime.

• Keep your bowels moving; when on the diet, your bowels should move 1 to 3 times a day. If you haven't had bowel movements for a whole day, you can do one of the following things; use the salt water flush; the salt has to be uniodized. Do this early in the morning with an empty stomach and expect to have bowel movements within 30 minutes. You can also use the MAG07 pills. Take 3 to 4 pills before you go to sleep and expect bowel movements in the morning. Bowel movements should however not be a problem with this diet. These are just precautionary measures.

• Detox family and friends; as you concentrate in detoxing your body, it might be necessary to detach yourself from family and friends that keep on discouraging you.

It is very normal to want to stop the process when you start. It something very new to your body and the normal mechanism is for it to resist. You might fall severally but what you do not need is people pushing you down. Encourage yourself and remember that the results are worth it.

• Expect to experience detox symptoms; the symptoms are not pleasant at all but they are bearable. It will be unfair for me to let you go into the diet process without letting you know that they will be there. We will discuss more on what they are and the things that you can do to deal with them.

Detox Symptoms

The severity of the detox symptoms will depend on how toxic you were in the first place. The signs are unpleasant but they are there for a short while. The symptoms that you might experience include:

• Headaches, pain and nausea; these effects are exaggerated if you decide to take coffee in the first few days. The headaches are more common but may be accompanied by physical aches and joint pains. At times, you may even feel nauseated.

• Irritability; not being able to eat some of your favorite foods as you are used to may be very boring. As a result, you may end up being very irritable.

• Cravings; there are specific foods that your body was used to especially meat, dairy products and sugar. For the first few days after you deprive your body of these foods, you will experience cravings. This will however go away after some time.

• Fatigue; cutting down on the food and detoxification in itself will drain you. You will feel fatigued most of the time and you might need more rest than you have been having.

• Flu-like symptoms; some people tend to get the feeling as if they are almost having a flu and will have muscle aches. To some, mucus discharge might be present too.

• Skin rashes; in the first days, it may be normal to experience skin rashes and even acne. This happens as the body tries to eliminate the toxins. As you keep on with the diet, the skin will get better.

At times, these symptoms may be very severe; if so, some of the things that you could do are:

1. Change the ratio of fruits to vegetables. You can start by having more fruits as you work your way to taking more vegetables. An acceptable ratio would be 70% of fruits

to 30% of vegetables. Adjust the ratios slowly as you move on.

2. Hydrate; in most cases, the headaches might be because of dehydration. During such cases, increasing your water intake may prove to be of great benefit.

3. Ease gradually into the food cleanse; starting with the full cleanse may be quite stressing for your body. Something that you could do is introducing it slowly until it fits in then start on it. You could start by doing away with your breakfast and morning snacks to accommodate the smoothies then continue with the next main meals.

Some Vegetables Used During Their Cleanse And Their Importance

You can use different vegetables in making your green smoothies. They all have different and important properties. That is the reason why it is advisable to alternate their use from week to week to be able to benefit from the whole range of their nutritional value. Some examples of these greens are:

• Arugula; it has a zippy, peppery flavor. It is rich in folic acid, vitamin A, C and K. It provides a boost for bone and brain health.

• Bok Choy; as the name suggests, its origin is Chinese. It is mild tasting and crunchy. It is rich in vitamins A, C, and calcium. It also has antioxidants.

• Beet greens; famous for improving vision, preventing Alzheimer and boosting the immune system. It is also rich in vitamin K.

• Collard greens; they are very similar to kale but with a much stronger taste. They are good in lowering cholesterol attributed to the fact that they have the ability to bind bile acids throughout the digestive tract.

• Dandelion Greens; these might look like weeds in your lawn. They are a great source of vitamin A and K. They are a great help in the digestion process and help with constipation issues. They actually act as a natural laxative.

• Chard; it has a beet-like taste but of a mild texture. In appearance, it is a green leafy vegetable, which has red stems, stalks and leaf veins. It is known to be very effective for cleansing the gut and preventing cancers.

• Kale; This vegetable lowers the risks that come with bladder, colon, breast, ovary, and prostate. It has ruffled leaf edges and is very rich in vitamin A, C, K.

• Spinach; almost everyone is in love with this vegetable. It is mild tasting and not as bitter as the others. It has high levels of omega 3s, vitamins A, C, E and K, calcium and magnesium. Most people make a point of starting with these.

• Parsley; famous for being able to control aging and regulating blood sugar levels. It is rich in antioxidants, minerals, vitamins, and fiber.

• Lettuce; it is popular from the time of ancient Egyptians. It is a good source of Vitamin C, K, A and folic acid. Be sure to get the dark green leaves, as they are the ones with the highest nutritional value.

• Mustard greens; these is the storehouse of phytonutrients which is famous for the prevention of a multitude of diseases. They are very effective in lowering cholesterol levels and providing riboflavin, niacin, magnesium, and iron.

• Turnip greens; they are flavorful but slightly bitter. They stand out for their ability in fighting off many of the cancerous cells.

Doing The 10 Day Green Smoothie Cleanse

We have come a long way in understanding the benefits of the green smoothie, the challenges that we expect to face and even some of the vegetables are great. By this time, you must be very ready to start on 'The 10 day green smoothie cleanse'. As you prepare for this, please remember the tips we have shared and the foods to include in your diet. I do not expect you to include the starchy vegetables like the sweet potatoes and carrots. Stick to the green leafy and add some fruits.

I also understand that there will be cravings but as we said, try to fight them off by ensuring you don't get too angry and you eat some health snacks that we had looked at earlier. When blending, remember to wash the fruits and vegetables since they have been exposed to pesticides in the fields. The water you use in the blending is also vital. Avoid using tap water and go for purified water.

Preparation

Get mentally prepared for the cleanse. Take your baseline measurements as well as a photo before you start. Purpose to begin each day by taking a few glasses of water, and then follow it up with detox tea. Remember to always stay rehydrated to avoid the severe symptoms of detoxification. Do not forget to buy fruits and veggies that will last you for the first five days. Once you start on the diet plan, you will feel very drained and shopping will not be something that you would want to participate in.

How to do the 10 day green smoothie cleanse

Under the 10 day green smoothie cleanse, there are two types of cleansing from which you can choose from. The cleansing can either be full or modified. For either cleanse you will have to avoid what we talked about earlier which include milk, cheese, refined sugar, liquor, beer, sodas, coffee, fried and processed food and refined carbs.

Full Cleanse

This consists of 3 smoothies, snacks and water/tea for the 10 days. It will provide the most weight loss benefits of between 10-15 pounds. It however needs you to be strong and committed to the process.

Summary

• Drink smoothies. For each day, you will need to drink 3 green smoothies. One will be for breakfast, the other lunch, and the last one for supper. It is also advisable to sip on the smoothie as the day progresses especially when you feel hungry. Do not forget to drink a smoothie or take a snack every 3-4 hours so that your metabolism is as it should. Each smoothie that you consume should contain approximately 12-16 ounces of liquid. Make an adequate amount of smoothie in the morning to last you the entire day and keep it refrigerated.

• Remember to snack; carry with you the recommended snacks that are apples, cucumbers, celery, carrots, peanut butter, unsalted nuts and hard-boiled eggs. Do not starve yourself.

• Drink water and detox tea; remember the desired amount of water per day you need to take. Also include herbal teas. Start with these two early in the morning to aid in the detox process by cleansing the kidneys, liver, and skin.

Modified cleanse

This consists of two green smoothies. One for breakfast and the other one for lunch. You could do one healthy meal for supper, snacks and water. The healthy meal may consist of a salad, sautéed vegetables, fish or chicken. Make the chicken either grilled or boiled. Weight loss might not be as much as with the full cleanse but it has tremendous health benefits. You can still expect to lose between 5-10 pounds in the 10 days. It is the best option if your goal is not mainly to lose weight but to detox.

Summary

• Drink smoothies and eat 1 healthy meal; each day, drink two green smoothies for breakfast and for lunch and eat one healthy meal for dinner. Each smoothie should contain 12-16 ounces of liquid. Just like in the full cleanse, prepare the smoothie in the morning to last you for the entire day.

• Eat snacks. You are still free to indulge in the healthy snacks just like the ones that we have discussed above. Do not overindulge though.

• Drink water and detox tea as stipulated above and make sure you do not become dehydrated. Take at least 8 glasses of water.

• Keep the bowel moving.

- Keep off the prohibited foods.

Losing Weight After The 10 Days

Getting to this point was the toughest part; once here, it is easier to keep the weight off and even lose some more pounds. You must be already feeling vibrant and happy and it should be your decision to remain that way. Engage in activities that will keep you healthy and nourished spiritually as well as physically. So how do you keep on losing weight and staying healthy?

Breaking the cleanse

The temptation that you might have is going back to fully eating what you feel like. This should not be the case. You do have the right to make yourself happy but we do not want to get back to where we were in the first place. So as you break off the cleansing, start by introducing a meal after the other. Maintain the smoothies to keep you healthy and full. The goal here is to make sure that you eat light and the portions must be acceptable. This is the only way that you will successfully continue losing weight.

Continuing to lose weight after the cleanse

The cleanse gives you a jumpstart of about 10-15 pounds to start your weight loss journey. From there, you should continue having a normal and healthy weight loss of about 1-2 pounds every week. There are foods that we are going to look into to ensure that you are able to achieve this. As you do this, remember to include proteins in every meal. The importance of proteins is that they help build your muscles and prevent muscle wasting. They also give you a feeling of fullness and prevent unnecessary overeating and food cravings.

Below are examples of 10 high protein meals.

• Chicken or lean steak in a Caesar salad

- Baked chicken with baked sweet potato and sautéed veggies

- Chicken stir-fry with brown rice

- Turkey chili

- Grilled salmon with a garden salad

- Grilled salmon with quinoa and veggies

- Grilled halibut with stir-fried veggies

- Lean steak with sweet potatoes and veggies

- Lean sirloin steak with lima beans

- Tuna on a garden salad

Let us look at some tips that will help you to continue losing weight even after the cleanse.

Tips on losing weight the healthy way

• Avoid empty calories; try to choose the foods that have been labeled to be rich in minerals, phytonutrients, fiber and vitamins. Keep off junk foods as most of them contain empty calories. You want to heal your body and maintain it in a healthy state.

• Eat a big salad everyday; this increases your vegetable intake and the nutritional value. Try the dark leafy vegetables.

• Avoid sugar, salt, and trans fat; these are known for causing weight gain. They also have no nutritional value. They are also associated with all the irritating digestive symptoms like bloating, swelling and fluid retention.

• Eat protein with every meal; we have gone over and over again about the importance of proteins. It goes without saying that it should be included in your diet.

• Limit the red meat to 2-3 times a week. This is because meat contains saturated fats that we are trying to limit. Strive to eat more of fish, poultry and chicken

• Buy organic food as much as possible; these are foods that do not have preservatives, additives, pesticides, or antibiotics. Fresh foods are less toxic as compared to the processed foods. Keep off them.

• Avoid starving yourself; the problem of getting yourself starved is the lack of control when you come across some food. Try to eat 4-5 meals a day. If you have three main meals, try to snack in between.

• Drink green tea; apart from green tea having many benefits like preventing diseases, it also helps with weight loss. It is also a good anti-oxidant, and comes in handy in preventing high blood pressure that has become a major problem. Some of the examples of these has been discussed above

• Drink more water; you can do this when you wake up, the times you feel hungry and with your meals too. Apart from helping in the detoxification, it gives you a feeling of fullness and helps reduce the cravings.

Best And Worst Foods When Losing Weight

Generally, there are foods that are considered to be very good when you are losing weight while others will keep on taking you back to square on. I find it necessary for you to know such kinds of food for they will guide your decision-making.

Meat

Eat; Tilapia, Trout, Tuna, Skinless Chicken, Lobster, Oysters, Sardines, Shrimp, Turkey breast, Crabmeat, Catfish.

Avoid; sausage, hot dogs, bacon, beef jerky, high fat meat like prime rib, pepperoni, salami.

Vegetables

Eat; all dark greens most have been mentioned above. Others include mushrooms, onions, olives, peas, tomatoes, yams, zucchini, Brussels, cauliflower.

Avoid; white potatoes, red potatoes, corn and plantains. Most vegetables are generally good for you.

Fruits

Eat; most of the fruits are healthy for you, but if you are trying to lose weight, you can specialize on most of the berries, lemons, limes, avocado, and passion.

Avoid; canned fruits and dried fruits. These are usually very high in sugar.

Grains

Eat; brown rice, coconut flour, oats, wild rice, barley, bulgur and quinoa

Avoid; white rice, white pasta, white bread, bagels, donuts and white flour

Dairy

Eat; egg white, almond milk, coconut milk, goat milk. oat milk, rice milk, non-dairy butter, eggs

Avoid; regular cow milk, cheese, cottage cheese, cream cheese, sour cream, yoghurt, powdered milk

Beans/Legumes:

Eat: Black-eye peas, Garbanzo beans/Chickpeas, Black beans, Green beans, Kidney beans, Fava beans, Lima beans, Navy beans, Lentils, White beans

Avoid; Dried beans, Refried beans

Nuts and Seeds:

Eat: Raw and Unsalted Nuts and Seeds: examples of such are chia seeds, walnuts, pecans, sunflower seeds, sesame seeds, pumpkin seeds, hemp seeds, Brazil nuts, almonds, macadamia nuts, hazelnuts, cedar nuts and cashews. The next best are roasted and unsalted nuts and seeds.

Avoid: Sugar-coated nuts and seeds

Oils:

Eat: Avocado oil, Flaxseed oil, Sesame oil, Coconut oil, Extra-virgin Olive oil, Fish oil,

Avoid; Bacon fat, vegetable oils, Chicken fat, Margarine, Hydrogenated oils (transfats)

Delicious Green Smoothie Recipes

Super Green

Makes: 32 fl. oz. – 4 servings
Time: 10 minutes

Ingredients:

3 cups orange juice
1 cup mango
1 ½ cups kale, chopped
4 celery stalks, trimmed
1 bunch parsley, fresh, chopped
1 bunch mint, fresh, chopped

Directions:

Place all ingredients in a food blender.

Process until smooth. This will only work if you have large blender, if not you can make the smoothie in batches.

Serve immediately.

Kale Blast

Serves: 32 fl. oz. – 4 servings
Time: 10 minutes

Ingredients:

1 ½ cups coconut water
1 avocado, peeled, stoned
1 cucumber, washed and peeled if want
1 lemon, washed and sliced
1 ½ cups kale, chopped
1 bunch cilantro, fresh, chopped
1-inch ginger, peeled

Directions:

In a food blender, place the ingredients, half of each.

Process until smooth.

Repeat with remaining ingredients and serve in chilled glass.

Spinach-Almond Milk Smoothie

Makes: 32 fl. oz. – 4 servings
Time: 10 minutes

Ingredients:

2 cups almond milk
2 cups packed spinach
1 avocado, peeled, stoned
1 pear, cored, sliced
2 teaspoons Chia seeds
½ cup water

Directions:

In a food blender, combine all ingredients.

If you have smaller blender, blend the ingredients in few batches or you can place all in one larger blender.

Pulse until the ingredients are smooth and blended thoroughly.

Serve immediately in chilled glasses.

Clean Smoothie

Makes: 32 fl. oz. - 4 servings
Time: 10 minutes

Ingredients:

2 apples, washed and cored
2 cups water
4 tablespoons lemon juice
2 celery stalks, trimmed
½ cup cilantro
1 ½ tablespoons Chia seeds
1 teaspoon cinnamon

Directions:

In a food blender place all ingredients.

Pulse all at once or make smoothie working
in batches.

Serve immediately in chilled glasses.

Spring Smoothie

Makes: 32 fl. oz. – 4 servings
Time: 12 minutes

Ingredients:

2 cups green tea, chilled
2 cups pineapple
2 cups cilantro
2 cups cucumber
2 ½ cups baby kale
2 tablespoons ginger, fresh grated
1 avocado
2 lemons, juiced and zested

Directions:

In a food blender combine all ingredients by order.

Pulse until smooth.

Serve in chilled glasses or with few ice cubes.

Ultimate Creamy Green Detox Smoothie

Makes: 32 fl. oz. - 4 servings
Time: 12 minutes

Ingredients:

14 oz. water or coconut water
1 orange, peeled
2 bananas, peeled, sliced
3 cups kale, chopped
1 lime, peeled
2 tablespoons chia seeds
1 tablespoon ginger, fresh grated

Directions:

Add all ingredients in food blender, except the kale.

Pulse few times until blended thoroughly.

Add the kale and pulse for additional 30-50 seconds.

Serve after.

Coconut Oil Detox Smoothie

Makes: 32 fl. oz. – 4 servings
Time: 10 minutes

Ingredients:

1 cup almond or coconut milk
2 tablespoons coconut oil, virgin, melted
2 cups ice
3 cups kale, chopped
1 ½ cucumbers
1 lime, peeled, sliced
4 celery stalks
1 apple, cored, sliced

Directions:

Place all ingredients in food blender.
If your blender is smaller, just divide the
ingredients in half. Pulse the ingredients
until you have smooth and thoroughly
blended drink.

Serve after.

Detox Goddess

Time: 32 fl. oz. – 4 servings
Time: 10 minutes

Ingredients:

2 green apples, cored
1 banana, peeled, sliced
2 cups water
2oz. romaine lettuce leaves
1 lemon, peeled
2 cups baby kale
1 cup ice cubes
1 bunch parsley, fresh, chopped
Stevia – to taste
2 tablespoons flax seeds, ground

Directions:

Place all ingredients in a food blender.

Process until smooth. If your blender is small, prepare the smoothie in batches.

Serve after.

Energy And Detox Smoothie

Makes: 32 fl. oz. – 4 servings
Time: 12 minutes

Ingredients:

2 cups spinach
1 cup ice cubes
1 cucumber, washed
2 green apples, cored
1 cup almond milk
1 tablespoon peanut butter, organic and smooth
2 teaspoons stevia

Directions:

Combine all ingredients in a blender.

Blend on high for 1 minute or until smooth.

Serve immediately.

Green Peach Smoothie

Makes: 32 fl. oz. – 4 servings
Time: 10 minutes

Ingredients:

2 cups coconut milk
3 cups baby spinach
2 cups peaches, sliced
2 oranges, peeled

Directions:

In a food blender combine all ingredients.

Process until smooth. Serve in chilled glasses.

Power Detox Smoothie

Makes: 32 fl. oz. – 4 servings
Time: 10 minutes

Ingredients:

2 cups water
2 pears
4 tablespoons lemon juice
1 cup celery, chopped
1 ½ cup cucumber, chopped
1 cup lettuce, romaine, chopped
1 cup spinach
1 tablespoon chia seeds
1-inch ginger, grated
¼ teaspoon cinnamon
¼ teaspoon turmeric
2 tablespoons mint, fresh, chopped
2 tablespoons parsley, fresh, chopped

Directions:

Place all ingredients in blender and blend until smooth.

Serve in chilled glass and if desired sweeten with stevia or honey.

Green Berry Smoothie

Makes: 32 fl. oz. - 4 servings
Time: 10 minutes

Ingredients:

2 cups blueberries, fresh
1 cup spinach
3 pcs cucumber
2 cups water
1 pcs avocado
2 tablespoons lime juice

Directions:

Combine ingredients in food blender.

Process on high until smooth and blended
thoroughly.

Serve in chilled glasses.

Date Green Smoothie

Makes: 32 fl. oz. – 4 servings
Time: 10 minutes

Ingredients:

2 cups coconut water
2 cups dandelion greens
2 ½ cups green grapes
1 lemon, peeled
8 dates, pitted
Stevia – to taste

Directions:

Place all the ingredients in food blender.

Pulse until smooth and blended thoroughly.

Serve after.

Kiwi Detox Smoothie

Makes: 32 fl. oz. – 4 servings
Time: 10 minutes

Ingredients:

4 pcs kiwi, peeled
2 cups water
2 tablespoons mint, chopped
2 cups romaine lettuce, chopped
2 celery stalks, trimmed, sliced
Stevia – to taste

Directions:

Combine all ingredients in food blender.

Process until smooth. Serve in chilled glass.

Mango Paradise

Makes: 32 fl. oz. – 4 servings
Time: 10 minutes

Ingredients:

1 cup mango, peeled, diced
2 cups coconut water
1 ½ cups beet greens, chopped
1 lime, peeled
1 cup ice
2 tablespoons mint
Honey- to taste

Directions:

Prepare the ingredients as described.

Place all ingredients in food blender.

Pulse until smooth and serve after.

Arugula Green Blast

Makes: 32 fl. oz. – 4 servings
Time: 10 minutes

Ingredients:

2 cups arugula
2 green apples, cored
1 cup water
1 cup orange juice
1 tablespoon ginger, fresh grated
1 lime, peeled
Stevia – to taste

Directions:

Prepare the ingredients as described.

Place all the ingredients in food blender and pulse until smooth.

Serve after.

Chard-Strawberry Smoothie

Makes: 32 fl. oz. - 4 servings
Time: 10 minutes

Ingredients:

2 ½ cups kale, chopped
1 cup strawberries
1 ½ cups water
½ cup Greek yogurt
1 cup pineapple, diced, fresh

Directions:

Place all the ingredients in high-power food blender.

Pulse until smooth and blended thoroughly.

Serve immediately.

Collard Greens Detox Smoothie

Makes: 32 fl. oz. – 4 servings
Time: 12 minutes

Ingredients:

2 cups water
3 cups collard greens, chopped
2 pcs grapefruit, pink
1 tablespoon honey
¼ cup mint

Directions:

Ina food blender combine all ingredients.

Pulse until smooth and blended thoroughly.

Serve in chilled glass.

Melon Green Paradise

Makes: 32 fl. oz. – 4 servings
Time: 10 minutes

Ingredients:

2 cups spinach
2 cup melon
2 cups coconut water
¼ cup pineapple juice
1 teaspoon cinnamon
1 teaspoon stevia

Directions:

Place all the ingredients in food blender.

Process until smooth.

Serve after.

Green Rice Delight

Makes: 32 fl. oz. – 4 servings
Time: 10 minutes

Ingredients:

2 cups rice milk
2 cups spinach, chopped
2 pcs bananas, sliced
1 avocado, peeled, stoned
2 tablespoons dates, chopped

Directions:

Prepare all ingredients as described.

Pop the ingredients in food blender and pulse until smooth.

Serve in chilled glass.

Conclusion

Going on a green smoothie cleanse is not easy but it is possible. With the right preparation and mindset, you will truly be able to start on it and be successful. Of great importance is to be aware of the detox symptoms so that you can deal with them adequately instead of giving up. Commit into doing this and experience the rewards.

www.ingramcontent.com/pod-product-compliance
Lightning Source LLC
Chambersburg PA
CBHW062117280526
45788CB00003B/1494